The Secret Benefits of Juice Therapy

The Secret Benefits of Juice Therapy

VIJAYA KUMAR

NEW DAWN PRESS, INC.
USA• UK• INDIA

NEW DAWN PRESS GROUP
Published by New Dawn Press Group
New Dawn Press, Inc., 244 South Randall Rd # 90, Elgin, IL 60123
e-mail: sales@newdawnpress.com

New Dawn Press, 2 Tintern Close, Slough, Berkshire, SL1-2TB, UK
e-mail: salesuk@newdawnpress.org

New Dawn Press (An Imprint of Sterling Publishers (P) Ltd)
A-59, Okhla Industrial Area, Phase-II, New Delhi-110020, India
e-mail: info@sterlingpublishers.com
www.sterlingpublishers.com

The Secret Benefits of Juice Therapy
© 2006, Sterling Publishers (P) Ltd
ISBN 978-1-84557-535-9
Reprint 2007

Contents

Contents

Introduction

For centuries, fruit and vegetable juices have been used for their therapeutic benefits. It not only reverses the degeneration of the body but also arrests the rate at which you age, and brings you seemingly boundless energy. Fresh juice enables you to easily assimilate useful nutrients in the body. Since enzymes, essential for digestion, get destroyed when food is cooked, there is all the more reason why fresh, raw produce should constitute at least half of your diet.

Hence, the consumption of fresh, raw vegetables and fruits prove to be more beneficial to our health than other food.

Essential Facts About Juices

Juices offer you the essential concentration of nutrients in the best proportion to nourish and synergise your body.

The juices of fresh fruits and vegetables are the richest sources of minerals, vitamins and enzymes.

The less the food is processed, the more it retains its active nutrients.

Always remember to have fresh produce, and extract the juice only when required, instead of storing it for days.

Avoid bottled, canned or frozen juices for these are usually preserved with chemicals, which destroy the healthy nutrients.

To add a wide variety of nutrient-rich beverages into one's diet, have juices.

Since fibre is essential for good health, it is recommended that juice intake should be complemented by a high-fibre diet.

It is always better to take fresh fruits and vegetables in the form of juices than depend on vitamin and mineral pills, because nutrients combined naturally in food, work much more effectively than in the pill form.

You may combine raw fruit and vegetable juices if you do not experience any adverse symptoms.

It is recommended that organically grown produce should be used more, as it is free from exposure to harmful sprays, like pesticides, herbicides and other toxic chemicals.

Several glasses of juice per day is recommended; ideally, two to four glasses, in addition to meals, provides good balance.

An equal proportion of vegetable and fruits juices are advisable.

You can introduce to your baby, aged between six and nine months, small amounts of juice.

While extracting juice, remove the skin of orange and grapefruit as they contain a toxic substance.

Similarly, apple seeds contain cyanide, and hence should be removed before extracting juice from an apple.

Avoid carrot leaves, as they too are believed to have toxins.

Before extracting juice, wash the produce well, removing damaged or unwanted portions.

Remove pits from fruits like apple, peach, plum, etc. You may retain the seeds of lemon, grapes, limes, etc., when extracting juice.

If you are fasting, always break the fast with a glass of fresh raw vegetable or fruit juice.

Juices of green leafy and yellow vegetables like spinach, carrot, yellow pumpkins contain vitamin A, riboflavin and iron.

Citrus fruits, tomato and raw cabbage provide ascorbic acid and iron, if taken in the form of fresh juice, or eaten raw.

Tender leaves and stems of vegetables contain alkalis.

Fresh fruit and vegetable juices cleanse and rejuvenate the human body.

Indispensable Nutrients

Raw fruits and vegetables are nature's way of giving us food good for health. Food is the 'fuel' that keeps the body in good working order and supplies energy for all activities.

No single natural food can supply all the elements that are required to make a diet that is nutritionally adequate, and hence combinations of various foods are required.

Food is composed of many different nutrients, each of which perform a different function in the body.

Carbohydrates
Carbohydrates form the bulk of the nutrients.

In the presence of sunlight and chlorophyll carbon dioxide and water react and combine to form carbohydrates.

In their natural, unrefined state, carbohydrates are an important source of energy and nutrition.

Carbohydrates are divided into three types: sugar, starch and fibre.

Sugar

It occurs naturally in certain foods, for example, fructose in fruits and lactose in milk. Refined sugar (sucrose) is an 'empty' food for it has no nutrients at all.

Starch

Starch is a tasteless white substance found in several foods, such as rice, cereals, bread, potatoes, etc. Since it tends to be bulky, it gives the stomach a feeling of fullness.

Fibre

Fibre is an indigestible carbohydrate that cannot be absorbed by the body.

Sometimes called roughage, fibre simply passes through the digestive tract, helping in reducing the risk of constipation and other diseases.

Fibre is beneficial for slimmers as, when consumed with liquid, it gives the stomach a feeling of fullness, so you end up eating less than usual.

The recommended daily fibre intake for adults is about 30 gm.

Good sources of fibre include grain cereals, wholemeal products, jacket potatoes, highly cooked vegetables, pulses and fruits with skin, for example, an apple before being peeled.

Protein
Protein is used for the building, maintenance and repair of body tissues.

Protein should constitute 10-15 per cent of your daily calorie intake.

Good sources of low-fat proteins include poultry, white fish, eggs, soya products, cottage cheese and yoghurt.

Other less-rich sources include cereals, bread, rice, potatoes and pulses.

Fats and oils

These have a higher calorific value than any other food, so their intake should be kept to a minimum in any diet.

Remember some foods have a 'hidden' fat content like cakes, biscuits, pastries, ice-cream, chocolate and meat.

Fats may be divided into saturates, monounsaturates, and polyunsaturates. All fats contain a mixture of the three, so they are labelled according to the type that predominates.

Saturated fats

Found in dairy products, like red meat, hard fats and coconut oil, saturated fats are not an essential part of the diet.

They are believed to cause an accumulation of cholesterol in the blood which coats the arteries and can lead to heart attack.

It is better to avoid saturated fats and minimise consumption of high cholesterol food such as egg yolk and liver.

Monounsaturated fats

These are present in olive oil, nuts and seeds, and should be consumed in preference to saturated fats.

Polyunsaturated fats

These are the only fats that the body needs as they contain two essential fatty acids that cannot be synthesised by the body.

Vitamins

These are chemical compounds that the human body needs in small amounts and are necessary for growth and health. There are two kinds of vitamins:

Fat-soluble vitamins are A, D, E and K, and are stored in the liver and fatty tissues.

Water-soluble vitamins, B-complex and C, cannot be stored for long, so adequate amount must be taken regularly.

Vitamin A

These are found in abundance in carrots, milk, butter, egg yolk, cheese, tomatoes, dark green vegetables, yellow and orange fruits, liver, halibut and cod liver oil.

Vitamin B-complex

Vitamin B$_1$ (Thiamin)
It is found in milk, beans, bacon, pork, liver, kidney, pulses, peanuts, oatmeal, flour, bread, brewer's yeast, wheat-germ and enriched breakfast cereals.

Vitamin B$_2$ (Riboflavin)
It is found in milk, yoghurt, cheese, liver, kidney, egg, bran, brewer's yeast and curd.

Vitamin B$_3$ (Niacin)
It is found in peanuts, wholemeal bread, brewer's yeast, meat, liver, coffee, beer, pulses, potatoes and enriched cereals.

Vitamin B$_6$ (Pyridoxine)
It is found in potatoes, leafy vegetables, fresh and dried fruits, nuts, cereals and whole grains.

Vitamin B$_{12}$
It is found in liver, heart, sardines, eggs, milk and cheese.

Folic Acid

It is found in liver, fish, avocados, green vegetables, wholemeal bread, eggs, bananas, oranges, bran, beetroot and peanuts.

Vitamin C

It is found in fresh fruits and vegetables, but can get drastically reduced by prolonged cooking or storage. Good sources include green raw cabbage, citrus fruits, guava, gooseberries, green and red peppers, sprouts and watermelons.

Vitamin D

It is produced by the action of sunlight on the skin. It is also found in herrings, salmon, sardines, mackerel, pilchards, egg yolks, margarine, butter and liver.

Vitamin E

It is found in dark green vegetables, wheat-germ, vegetable oils, whole grains, nuts and eggs.

Vitamin K

It is found in leafy vegetables, yoghurt and egg yolk.

Minerals

These are needed for the growth and maintenance of body structures. They are found in the form of calcium, iodine, iron, magnesium, phosphorus, potassium, sodium and zinc.

Calcium

It is found in dairy products, sardines, soya beans, broccoli, peanuts and white bread.

It is essential for growth and formation of bones.

Iodine

It is found in milk, eggs, meat, seafood and vegetables.

Iron

Menstruating women and girls need a good supply of iron to lessen the chances of becoming anaemic.

It is found in liver, kidney, beef, wholemeal bread, potatoes, watercress, dried apricots and soya sauce.

Magnesium

Vegetables and grains are rich sources of magnesium.

Phosphorus

It is commonly found in nuts, eggs, soya and whole grains.

Potassium

It is found in milk, vegetables and fruits.

Sodium

It is found in most vegetables, often added as salt.

Zinc

It is found in milk, hard cheese, wholemeal bread, meat and oysters.

Water

It is essential for every bodily process, either taken in its pure form or in the form of tea, coffee or low-calorie drinks.

Excess liquid is simply expelled in urine, flushing the body of its toxins.

Benefits of Juice

Research shows that people living on natural foods like raw fruits and vegetables thrive best – without an ailment in the body.

Fruit and vegetable juice therapy is very effective, as it removes the flaws from the body from their roots. Unlike drugs, it has no side effects, and is not known to damage any part of the body.

It does not result in any adverse reaction, mentally or physically.

Notwithstanding these, vegetables and fruits are cheaper than medicines.

Raw fruit and vegetable juice helps in detoxifying the body. Juice can be taken at any hour during the day or night. Juice helps to enhance ones energy level, relieve fatigue, and bolster up sagging spirits. They are health-giving, life-giving and youth-giving essential foods. One of the secrets of maintaining a youthful look is the continuous and persistent practice of getting the liquid extract of fruits and vegetables.

Juices bring a sparkle to the eyes, colour to the lips, and a spring to the step by revitalising the bloodstream. The most gratifying revelation by researchers is that people stricken with serious disorders like cancer, heart attack, etc., could become strong and robust with the intake of juices.

One's sluggish and tired nerves get revived, while glands and organs get rejuvenated with fruit and vegetable juices. A high-raw diet, in the form of juices, can not only reverse the bodily degeneration, but also make you feel emotionally better.

We derive our energy from plants that, in turn, get energised by the sun during the process of photosynthesis. The vital enzymes, vitamins and minerals that our body requires can be procured from these plants which absorb them from the rich soils. The cells in our body, in turn, absorb all these plant-derived essential nutrients.

Juices are rich in nutrients and, hence, make the best diet supplements. Water, minerals, vitamins, enzymes, etc., along with pigments, work harmoniously and synergistically to enable your body to heal, maintain good health and stay free of diseases.

Juices as Cure for Various Disorders

The dietary recommendations in this chapter will help the cells get nourished and thus progress towards healing and good health. These recommendations should be followed only to supplement your physicians suggestions.

All the suggestions for recipes and juicing will be effective only when incorporated with a total diet scheme.

Acne
This is an inflammation of the oil glands just beneath the surface of the skin, causing pimples, blackheads, whiteheads, and in extreme cases, infected cysts and scarred skin.

Ginger juice

    ¼ inch ginger

    4-5 carrots

    ½ apple, seeded

- Extract the juice from the above ingredients, mix well.
- Apart from being an effective detoxifier, ginger also freshens up ones skin as it is a good source of zinc.
- Cucumber prevents sunstroke, and is a good antidote for acne.
- Apple is high in carbohydrates, chromium and an excellent source of cellulose that acts against acne and pimples.

Aging

Aging is the process of growing old during which changes occur in the body as the result of passing time.

Fruity shake

    2 pineapple slices

    ½ cucumber

    ½ apple, seeded

- Run all these in a juicer.
- Pineapple is a good source of vitamin C, iron and essential minerals which act as tonic and rejuvenator.
- Apple is a good source of bioflavonoid that prevents free radical damage.
- You may also add black currant juice to your diet.
- Cabbage, yoghurt and olive oil are all said to increase longevity and slow down the aging process, and hence should be included in your diet.
- Use of thyme and lavender in dishes is also beneficial.
- High-fibre diet that includes oat and rice bran is recommended.

Allergies

Allergies are reactions to certain substances called allergens.

Red cocktail

¼ inch ginger piece

1 beetroot

½ apple, seeded

4 carrots

- Run all these through a juicer and mix well.
- Ginger is a good source of zinc which is important in healing of wounds, inflammation control and tissue regeneration.
- Apple is a good source of chromium that improves glucose tolerance levels and enhances insulin sensitivity.
- Carrots are a good source of beta-carotene, an antioxidant which helps in allergies.

Alopecia

It is a medical term for baldness where loss of hair mostly occurs on the scalp, but sometimes other parts of the body are also involved.

Parsley-spinach blend

A handful of parsley

A handful of spinach

4-5 carrots

2 stalks celery

- Extract their juice and mix well.

- Parsley is a good source of vitamin C that helps improve circulation in the scalp.
- Use of spinach, cabbage, legumes and eggs enhances hair growth.

Alzheimer's disease

This disease, resembling senile dementia, is characterised by loss of memory, lack of concentration, difficulties in communicating, severe mood swings, changes in personality, and inability to focus on day-to-day happenings.

Fruity punch

　　1 medium bunch of grapes
　　½ apple, seeded
　　¼ lemon
　　1 wedge of watermelon

- Run each through a juicer and mix well.
- Grapes and lemon are good sources of bioflavonoids, enhance vitamin C's effectiveness and help in blood circulation.
- Foods containing free radicals and some kinds of cheese that may be contaminated with aluminium should be avoided.

Amnesia

It is loss of memory. The loss can be of a great portion of one's memory, or partial, for example, an inability to remember names, colours or dates.

Green tonic

> A handful of parsley
> A handful of spinach
> 2 carrots
> 1 stalk of celery

- Extract the juice, and mix well.
- These are all rich in riboflavin, carotene, folate, iron and vitamin C, all of which are known to dramatically clear a foggy head.

Anaemia

It is a disorder of the blood in which the red cells are inadequate in number or have less haemoglobin than normal.

Iron booster

> Leaves of 3 beetroots
> 3-5 carrots
> ½ green pepper
> ½ apple, seeded

- Extract the juice from each, and mix well.
- Beetroot leaves and carrots are good sources of iron that help in enriching the blood.
- Green pepper is a source of vitamin C that helps in the absorption of iron in the body.
- You may also include beans, dried apricots, raisins, almonds and shellfish.

Anxiety

It is a feeling of intense worry or fear in the absence of obvious danger, which may cause tension and fatigue, and in extreme cases, profuse sweating and even irregular beating of the heart.

Fruity special

    1 cup strawberries

    ½ pear

    1 ripe banana

    1 tbsp brewer's yeast

- Run through a juicer, and mix well.
- Strawberry, rich in vitamin C, is an antioxidant, and so helps protect the body during stressful situations.

- Banana, rich in potassium, replenishes the body with this vital nutrient.
- Pears are rich in various vitamins and minerals that relieve stress.

Arthritis

It is a disease of the joints, wherein the patients suffer pain, stiffness and swelling in the joints.

Vegetable special

3 broccoli flowerets

2 tomatoes

2 stalks of celery

½ green pepper

1 clove of garlic

- Run each through the juicer, and mix well before use.
- Broccoli is a good source of pantothenic acid that helps in alleviating the pain associated with arthritis.
- Vitamin A, B and C, found in tomatoes, are beneficial in arthritis.
- Include whole grains, legumes, nuts, fruits and vegetables to supplement the diet.

Asthma

It is a disorder of the bronchial tubes, causing difficulty in breathing.

Energy greens

> A handful of spinach
> A handful of parsley
> 2 stalks of celery
> 4-5 carrots
> 1 clove of garlic

- Run the greens, and then the carrots, through the juicer.
- Spinach is a good source of vitamin B_6 that alleviates the frequency and severity of wheezing and asthma attacks.
- Parsley, rich in vitamin C, acts as a good defence against bronchial constriction.
- Garlic, containing selenium, inhibits the formation of inflammatory compounds.
- Celery is a good source of sodium that helps in maintaining chemical balance in the body.
- Generous helpings of onion and garlic in your diet ward off the enzyme responsible for inflammation of the bronchi.

Atherosclerosis

It is a condition in which deposits of fatty substances form inside an artery and obstruct the flow of blood.

Calcium-rich drink

> ¼ inch ginger
>
> 4-5 carrots
>
> A handful of parsley

- Run the carrot and ginger, followed by the greens, through a juicer, and mix well.
- Parsley and turnip greens provide the calcium essential for lowering cholesterol and triglycerides for preventing blood clots.
- Carrots and ginger are rich in copper which helps in reducing the cholesterol level in the blood.
- Garlic, ginger and onion should also be included in your diet.
- Hayseed oil, cold-water fish and fish oil are high in omega-3 fatty acids that are excellent for the prevention and care of atherosclerosis.

Backache

Pain in the back can be a symptom of various disorders – a strain, bad posture, a slipped disc, obesity, kidney disease, gall bladder infection or pregnancy.

Vitamin-rich drink

> 2 lettuce leaves
>
> A small wedge of cabbage
>
> 3 broccoli flowerets
>
> A handful of spinach
>
> 4-5 carrots
>
> ½ apple, seeded

- Run them through the juicer, separately, and mix well.
- The broccoli, lettuce, cabbage and spinach are rich sources of vitamin K, which help in reducing backache.
- Carrots are rich in copper, which is effective in controlling backache.
- Apple contains antibacterial compounds and helps in easing the pain.

Bronchitis

Strictly speaking, bronchitis is the inflammation of the bronchial tubes, affecting the air passage of the nose, throat and larynx and often the bronchioles.

Ginger tonic

> 2 inch ginger piece
> ¼ lemon
> 1 glass water
> 1 stick cinnamon
> 4-5 cloves
> A dash of cardamom

- Extract the juice from ginger and lemon. Add to water along with the other ingredients, and gently simmer.
- Ginger, a good source of zinc, promotes a healthy immune system.
- Lemon is a source of bioflavonoids which help in the absorption of vitamin C.
- Honey can be added to the tonic, as it is effective during the acute phase.

Bruise

A bruise is a concussion, which is a surface discolouration and swelling resulting from a blow or pressure.

Fruity concoction

>   1 large bunch grapes
>   2 apples, seeded
>   1 wedge of lemon
>   2-3 oranges, peeled

- Run each through a blender, and mix well.
- Grapes, lemon and oranges are good sources of bioflavonoids which, along with vitamin C, helps in preventing easy bruising.

Bursitis

This is a painful inflammation of the bruise where there is an accumulation of an abnormal amount of fluid, and the brusal sac becomes swollen.

Fruit cocktail

>   1 orange, peeled
>   ½ apple, seeded

1 small bunch grapes

1 slice pineapple

- Run each of the fruits mentioned through a juicer, separately, and combine the juices.
- The grapes and orange, rich in bioflavonoids, helps in stabilising collagen structures, and in reducing inflammation.
- Pineapple is a rich source of the enzyme bromelain, which is an effective anti-inflammatory agent.

Candidiasis

Candidiasis is an infection of mainly the gastrointestinal tract, nervous, endocrine and immune systems, during which there is chronic fatigue, low energy and malaise.

Mineral-rich juice

A handful of parsley

1 beet top

5 carrots

1 clove of garlic

3 stalks of celery

- Run these through a juicer, and mix well.

- Spinach is a source of vitamin B_6, which helps in the production of hydrochloric acid, and strengthens the immune system.
- Garlic contains selenium that enhances the immune system.
- Parsley and beet green are rich in iron, which is essential for producing energy, and for a healthy immune system.

Cataract

This is a clouded condition of the lens of the eye, which causes blurred vision, generally developed in elderly people.

Greens soup
    A handful of parsley
    A handful of spinach
    2 carrots
    ¼ inch ginger piece
    2-3 cloves of garlic
- Run them through the juicer, and mix well.
- Parsley and spinach are rich sources of beta-carotene, which protects the lenses of the eyes from light-induced damage.

- Garlic is a good source of vitamin B, that is essential in intracellular eye metabolism.

- Spinach contains vitamin B_2 and E, known to act against cataract and protect eyes from the damage caused by free radicals, respectively.

- Spinach and carrot are good sources of manganese which arrests cataract growth while parsley, with vitamin C, stops its progression.

- Garlic, with selenium in it, helps in preventing damage caused by free radicals.

- Carrot and garlic are sources of copper which aids in stopping and reversing cataract growth.

- Parsley, garlic and carrots contain zinc which helps in warding off the onset of cataract.

- Take plenty of legumes like beans, lentils and split peas.

- Eat a substantial quantity of green, red and yellow vegetables and fruits that are rich in vitamin C and beta-carotene.

- Also supplement your diet with nuts, whole grains and wheat-germ, which are good sources of vitamin E.

Cellulitis

It is an infection of the skin, which gives it a hard, red and shiny appearance.

Orange juice

    3 oranges, peeled

- Run the orange segments through a juicer.
- Orange is a good source of bioflavonoids which work with vitamin C in keeping the skin clear of blemishes.
- High-fibre foods like oats, whole grains, legumes, vegetables and fruits are also helpful for a clear skin.

Colitis

Colitis is the inflammation of the colon, the large intestine, which could be ulcerative.

Carotene-rich drink

    A handful of parsley
    A handful of spinach
    4-5 carrots
    ½ apple, seeded

- Run each through a juicer, and mix well.
- All the ingredients are rich sources of beta-carotene, which is necessary for tissue repair.
- Aloe vera juice can also be consumed for healing the mucosa of the intestine.
- A high-fibre diet containing brown rice, legumes, vegetables and fruits is recommended.
- Papaya is also good for colitis.

Common cold

This is an infectious disease of the respiratory system, particularly the nose, throat and bronchi.

Saucy juice

> 4 tomatoes
> ½ cucumber
> ¼ green pepper
> 1 clove of garlic
> 2 stalks of celery
> A dash of tabasco sauce

- Extract juices from all the vegetables, and add the sauce, stirring well.

- Tomatoes contain bioflavonoids that have antibacterial action.
- Cucumber helps in flushing away the toxins, for it has a diuretic effect.
- Green pepper is a rich source of vitamin C, which has an antibacterial and antiviral action.
- Garlic is a good source of zinc which has an antiviral property.
- Green juices, vegetables, soups and broth, herbal tea and ginger tea are also beneficial.
- A generous amount of onions and garlic intake is also a remedial measure.

Constipation

Constipation is difficulty in clearing of the bowel, for the waste material becomes compact and hard, making it painful to evacuate.

Cleansing drink

    handful of spinach
    2 beetroot tops
    1 clove of garlic
- Extract the juices and mix well.

- Spinach and beet greens are rich in folic acid that help in clearing the bowel.
- Garlic contains thiamin, which too helps in bowel evacuation.
- Prune, pear and apple have a laxative effect.
- Increase your intake of fresh fruits and vegetables, nuts, seeds, legumes and whole grains.

Crohn's disease

It is a severe inflammation of the intestine (also known as ileitis), and results in attacks of diarrhoea alternating with constipation, poor appetite and loss of weight.

Green cocktail

> 3 beet tops
> A handful of parsley
> A handful of spinach
> 4 carrots
> 1 turnip top

- Extract the juices and mix well.
- Beet greens and spinach contain folic acid that helps in absorption of nutrients.

- Carrots, parsley and spinach have beta-carotene that the body converts into vitamin A.
- Parsley is a good source of vitamin C. Turnip greens, having vitamin K, prevents internal bleeding.
- Parsley and beet greens are sources of calcium which helps in regulating the acid-base balance of the body.
- But greens, spinach and parsley contain magnesium, which helps in relaxing the muscles.
- Parsley and carrots are sources of zinc that aids in healing, inflammation control and tissue regeneration.

Cramps

Cramp is a sharp, stitch-like pain, which generally affects a group of muscles, and may come on suddenly during exercising in the cold, or trouble particularly the elderly people in bed during the night.

Carrot drink

> 5 carrots
>
> A handful of parsley
>
> 1 clove of garlic

- Run these through a juicer, and blend well.
- Carrots are a good source of potassium and calcium that control the chemical balance of the body.
- They are also rich in vitamin E that improves blood circulation.
- Parsley is a good source of magnesium that controls the chemical balance of the body.
- Drink plenty of water, and always dilute fruit juices, like grapes, lime, orange or blackberries with water.

Cystitis

It is an infection and inflammation of the urinary bladder.

Ginger concoction

> ¼ inch ginger piece
>
> 1 apple, seeded
>
> 1 carrot
>
> ½ lemon

- Extract the juices, and mix well.
- Carrot is rich in betacarotene which helps strengthen the immune system, and protects against infection.
- Lemon has bioflavonoids which have an antibacterial effect, and help in the absorption of vitamin C.
- Ginger, containing zinc, promotes a healthy immune system.
- Pomegranate juice mixed with water is good to counter cystitis.
- A generous amount of garlic and onions should be included in your diet.

Cancer

Cancer is one of the several diseases that result when the process of cell division, gets out of control and leads to the development of malignant cells.

Special cocktail

4 carrots

A handful of parsley

A handful of spinach

        1 clove of garlic

        1 turnip top

        1 potato

- Run all the ingredients through a juicer, and mix well.
- Carrots, parsley and spinach provide beta-carotene that inhibits the rapid growth of new cancer cells.
- Parsley also converts free radicals to harmless waste, and detoxifies carcinogenic compounds.
- Spinach and carrots are rich in vitamin E, which helps in arresting the growth of tumour.
- Garlic and turnip greens are rich sources of selenium that helps in protecting cell membranes, and strengthening the immune system.
- Turnip greens and parsley contain calcium, which helps in preventing colon cancer.
- Parsley, garlic and spinach, rich in potassium, are effective in arresting the growth of cancer cells.

- Potato and spinach are good sources of chromium that inhibits the growth of new cancer cells.

Depression

This is the state of feeling dejected or low in spirits, and may be considered as an occupational disorder.

Green broth

> 3 broccoli flowerets
> 1 clove garlic
> 4-5 carrots
> 1 beet green
> ½ green pepper

- Extract the juices, and mix well.
- Broccoli and beet greens are rich in riboflavin which helps in keeping the body healthy.
- Green pepper and broccoli contain vitamin C, that helps fight depression.
- Broccoli, a good source of calcium, may be effective for those undergoing postmenopausal and postpartum depression.
- Beet greens and garlic have magnesium, and garlic and carrots have potassium, both

minerals help one to get out of a depressive mood.

- High protein foods, like fish and legumes are recommended.
- Foods high in complex carbohydrates – raw fruits and vegetables, legumes, whole grains – are also beneficial in fighting depression.

Diabetes mellitus

This is a disorder in which the body is unable to control the use of sugar as a source of energy.

Effective cocktail

A handful of spinach

A handful of parsley

4 carrots

½ apple, seeded

- Extract the juices, and mix well.
- Spinach contains vitamin B_6, vitamin E, chromium and magnesium, which are helpful in significantly alleviating the disease.
- Carrots are rich in vitamin E, while apple is rich in chromium.

- Generous consumption of garlic, onions, raw food and raw vegetable juices is found to be highly beneficial for diabetics.

Diarrhoea

This is a frequent and excessive discharge of water from the bowel, the danger lying in excessive loss of water.

Cabbage cocktail

¼ cabbage

A little spinach

2 tomatoes

1 carrot

- Run through a juicer, and mix well.
- All the ingredients are rich sources of potassium, which can be lost excessively in diarrhoea.
- Spinach is rich in folic acid that may be helpful in chronic diarrhoea.
- Spinach and carrot are also good sources of organic sodium and spinach is also rich in magnesium, both of these minerals need to be replenished during diarrhoea.

- Fresh juices and plenty of fluids should be consumed.
- Banana, rice, apple and tea are a good remedy for upset stomach and diarrhoea.

Diverticulitis
This is an abnormal condition of the large intestine (colon) in which the movement of the hard faeces causes the colon to thicken.

Lettuce cocktail
> 3 lettuce leaves
> 3 carrots
> A handful of parsley
> 2 tomatoes

- Run these through a juicer, and blend well.
- Lettuce is a good source of vitamin K, which prevents internal bleeding.
- Carrots and parsley are rich in beta-carotene that has a healing effect on the intestinal mucosa.

- A high-fibre diet, containing unprocessed bran, brown rice, whole grain cereals, brown bread, fruits and vegetables, is recommended.

Eczema

This is a skin condition characterised by a red, itching rash and blisters.

Cleansing juice

> A handful of parsley
> A handful of spinach
> 4 carrots
> ½ cucumber
> ¼ inch ginger piece

- Extract the juices, and mix well.
- Carrots and spinach are rich in beta-carotene, which is required to avoid the skin being vulnerable to thickening.
- Ginger, parsley and carrots consist of zinc which may be beneficial.
- Cucumber soothes the skin.
- Increase your consumption of cold-water fish and oats.

Epilepsy

This is a disorder of the nervous system in which there may be periodic loss of consciousness accompanied by convulsive seizures.

Vegetable cocktail

> A handful of spinach
>
> 2 beat tops
>
> 3 carrots
>
> 1 clove garlic
>
> ½ cup cabbage
>
> 1 sweet potato

- Extract the juices, and blend well.
- Spinach and beet greens contain folic acid which is beneficial.
- Parsley has vitamin C that helps in destroying free radicals.
- Lemon is a source of bioflavonoids that prevents damage caused by free radicals.
- Spinach and carrots contain vitamin E that improves blood circulation and tissue repair.
- Garlic, a source of selenium, helps the body detoxify.

Fatigue

It is a feeling of tiredness, which can range from slight to severe, and in the latter case it is exhaustion.

Rejuvenating drink

A handful of spinach
2 carrots
½ green pepper
2 broccoli flowerets
1 clove of garlic
¼ inch ginger

- Extract the juices, and mix well.
- Spinach, garlic, ginger and carrots are good sources of zinc, selenium and B complex vitamins that enhance the immune function and increase energy levels.
- Carrots and spinach are rich sources of beta-carotene that helps in protecting against toxins.
- Green pepper and broccoli consist of vitamin C that helps in the functioning of the adrenal glands, has antiviral effects and strengthens the immune system.

- Broccoli, rich in pantothenic acid, helps in easing stress from the body.
- Consume foods high in omega-3 fatty acids like mackerel, sardines, tuna, etc.

Gingivitis

This is an inflammation of the gums that begins around the teeth and causes bleeding, eventually leading to permanent damage to the gums and teeth, if left untreated.

Mint tonic

A handful of mint

1 tomato

¼ inch ginger

1 glass of soda

- Extract the juice from the ingredients. Add soda just before drinking.
- All the ingredients are rich in bioflavonoids which help in reducing inflammation and stabilising the collagen structures.
- Eating a high-fibre diet helps in increasing the secretion of saliva, which has a protective effect.

Gout

In this disease, the chemical processes in the body are upset, leading to the production of abnormally large amounts of uric acid.

Strawberry juice

    12 strawberries

    1 apple

    A few cherries

- Extract the juice, and mix well.
- Strawberries and cherries contain vitamin C, which is known to lower serum uric acid, or help to neutralise it.
- Apple is a source of chromium that helps in regulating the glucose metabolism and preventing attacks of gout.

Headache

The blood vessels in the brain are interlaced with many nerves, and it is in these nerves that headache originates, may be due to tension, migraine, sinusitis, common cold, influenza, allergies, eye strain, etc.

Beneficial drink

    1 clove of garlic

    A handful of parsley

    4 carrots

    ¼ inch ginger

- Extract the juices, and mix well.
- Garlic and parsley are good sources of magnesium that help in relaxing the muscles.
- Ginger and garlic, rich in magnesium, help in inhibiting blood clotting and soothing the nerves.
- Consume generous helpings of cold-water fish like sardines, salmon, mackerel and tuna.

Herpes

It is an inflammation of the skin accompanied by the formation of clusters of small blisters and can be either herpes simplex (commonly known as cold sore) and herpes zoster or shingles.

Berry-ginger cocktail

    1 bunch of green grapes

    1 cup blackberries

    1 inch ginger piece

- Extract the juice, mix well and serve cold.
- The berries and grapes are good sources of polyphenols that help in inactivating the viruses in the body.
- Ginger contains zinc that strengthens the immune system.
- Consume generously all seafood, eggs, potatoes and dairy products.

Hypertension

It is the medical term for the disease commonly known as high blood pressure. High blood pressure is not only a serious condition by itself, but it is also the leading cause of heart attacks, strokes, and kidney failure.

Fruit shake

    1 cup of strawberries

    1 banana

    ½ apple, seeded

    ¼ cantaloupe or musk melon

- Extract juices, and mix well.
- Strawberry is a source of vitamin C, which helps in lowering the blood pressure.

- Cantaloupe and bananas are good sources of potassium, which is beneficial to those suffering from hypertension.
- Consume onions and garlic generously which help in lowering cholesterol, and thinning the blood, apart from lowering blood pressure.

Hypoglycemia

This is an abnormally low level of glucose in the blood, generally due to an excess of the hormone insulin.

Healthy tonic

> 3 lettuce leaves
>
> 4 carrots
>
> A handful of beans
>
> 2 brussels sprouts

- Extract the juices, and blend them well.
- Lettuce leaves are a good source of chromium which helps regulate the effects of insulin in glucose metabolism.
- Beans and brussels sprouts are rich in manganese which helps in the metabolism of glucose.

- Consume foods rich in complex carbohydrates and soluble fibres such as oats, beans and lentils.
- Include cinnamon, cloves, bay leaves and turmeric liberally.

Indigestion

This is a nonmedical term used vaguely, for almost any kind of disturbance in the digestive system, like stomach ache, upset stomach, nausea, vomiting, cramp, constipation, diarrhoea, etc.

Fruity shake

½ orange, peeled
½ lemon
½ papaya, peeled
½ banana
¼ pineapple

- Run through a juicer, and blend well.
- Pineapple is the only source of the enzyme bromelain, which is a protein-digesting enzyme.
- Papaya contains the enzyme papain, which is a protein-digester, and is an active blood

clotting agent also having vitamin B and C.

- Lemon and banana are appetite stimulants and protect the stomach from acids.
- Cabbage juice has ulcer-healing property, and hence can be taken once a day.

Insomnia
It is the inability to fall asleep or sleep restfully.

Nerve soother

> 1 broccoli floweret
>
> 3 carrots
>
> A handful of parsley
>
> A handful of spinach
>
> 1 stalk of celery

- Extract the juices, and blend well.
- Broccoli, spinach, carrots and parsley are good sources of niacin, vitamin B_6 and magnesium which converts the amino acid tryptophan into the sleep-inducing chemical, serotonin.
- Broccoli contains calcium that aids in muscle relaxation.

- Celery helps in soothing the nerves and relaxing the muscles.

Liver spots

It is also known as age spots, and is a harmless discolouration on the skin, medically known as chloasma.

Complexion tonic

    1 grapefruit, peeled

    1 apple, seeded

    4 cherries

    8 grapes

- Extract the juices, and blend well.
- All these fruits are rich in bioflavonoids that help in repairing tissues.
- Intake of beet juice detoxifies the liver.

Menopausal problems

Menopause is the period during which menstruation becomes irregular and finally ceases, and various problems may be experienced, like hot flushes, irritability, insomnia, dizziness and depression.

Healing tonic

> A handful of parsley
> ¼ head of cabbage
> A handful of spinach
> 1 stalk of celery

- Run through a juicer, and blend well.
- Cabbage contains bioflavonoids that helps reduce the symptoms of menopause.
- Spinach is rich in vitamin E that helps in reducing hot flushes.
- Parsley is an excellent source of calcium and magnesium, which are necessary in preventing osteoporosis.
- Soya foods contain plant oestrogens that supplement the oestrogens produced by the ovaries.

Menstrual problems

Menstruation is the periodic bleeding from the uterus in women of childbearing age; the problems may be depression, emotional tension, headache, puffiness of the abdomen, skin and other parts of the body, excessive, prolonged or painful menstruation.

Fruity concoction
¼ pineapple
½ cup grapes
6 cherries
½ apple, seeded
1 ripe banana

- Extract the juices and pulp, and blend well.
- Pineapple is a good source of bromelain that has anti-inflammatory properties, and relaxes the muscles.
- Cherries and grapes are rich in riboflavonoids which strengthen capillaries, reduce bleeding and increase the absorption of iron.
- Take plenty of parsley and garlic that contains magnesium, which relieves uterine muscle spasms.
- Cabbage, turnip greens and broccoli help in reducing excessive bleeding.

Nausea

This is a feeling of discomfort or queasiness in the stomach, which is usually relieved by vomiting.

Ginger tonic

> 2 inch ginger piece
> ¼ lemon
> A small handful of spinach
> 1 bunch of green grapes

- Run these through a juicer, and mix well.
- Ginger helps in relieving seasickness, motion sickness, and morning sickness.
- Lime controls nausea.
- Spinach contains vitamin B_6 that helps in relieving nausea.
- Grapes give freshness to the mouth.

Obesity

This is a condition of being overweight, with excessive accumulation of fat in various parts of the body.

Cool cucumber drink

> 2 tomatoes
> 1 cucumber
> 2 stalks of celery
> 2 mint leaves for garnish

- Juice the tomatoes and freeze in ice-cube tray. Juice the cucumber and celery, and pour into a tall glass, adding the tomato cubes and garnish.
- Tomatoes are rich in vitamin A, B and C. They help in digestion and keeping the blood alkaline.
- Cucumber and celery aid in digestion, and help to burn calories.

Premenstrual tension

This is mental and physical distress before menstruation, during which there is general oedema, nervousness, irritability, depression, frequent headaches and pain in the breasts.

Protein-rich shake

    3 pineapple slices

    1 ripe banana

    1 orange, peeled

    2 inch sliced watermelon

    ½ cup soya milk

- Extract the juices and pulp, and blend well with soya milk.

- Pineapple, a source of bromelain, relaxes the muscles.
- Watermelon is a natural diuretic that helps to flush out the toxins in the body.
- Soya milk is rich in protein that helps in enhancing the haemoglobin level.
- Banana is rich in potassium and orange in bioflavonoids, both of which help in the relaxation of muscles and in blood circulation.

Prostatitis

Prostatitis is inflammation or enlargement of the prostate gland, which may occur as a result of an infection in the urinary tract.

Ginger ale

    ¼ inch ginger piece
    1 wedge of lemon
    1 bunch of green grapes
    Mineral water or soda

- Extract the juices, and add mineral water/ soda just before consuming.
- Ginger is a very good source of zinc that helps in reducing the size of the prostate gland.

- Grapes sooth the nerves and helps to relax the muscles.
- Also include in your diet, split peas, whole grains, lima beans and pumpkin seeds.

Psoriasis

It is a skin disease characterised by itchy, red patches that become covered with loose, silvery scales.

Spicy tonic

> ¼ pineapple
> ½ papaya
> ¼ inch ginger
> ½ apple, seeded
> ½ orange
> 1 carrot

- Extract the juice, and blend well.
- Carrot contains the essential mineral zinc which is necessary for the absorption of linoleic acid for healthy skin.
- Orange is a good source of selenium that helps in decreasing the formation of inflammatory compounds.

- Pineapple and papaya contain the enzyme bromelain which helps in protein digestion.
- Ginger is a natural anti-inflammatory agent.
- A high-fibre diet helps bind toxins in the bowel and flush them out.
- Consumption of salmon, herring and mackerel arrests skin inflammation.

Raynaud's disease

This is a disease of the arteries, affecting the feet, hands and, occasionally, nose and ears, during which the blood supply to these areas is temporarily cut off, leading to numbness, followed by severe pain when the circulation is restored.

Spicy greens

A handful of parsley

A handful of spinach

1 carrot

1 stalk of celery

1 clove of garlic

½ onion

- Extract the juices, and blend well.

- The greens are an excellent source of vitamin B-complex and chlorophyll that improves blood circulation.
- Garlic and onion are rich in geranium that enhances oxygen supply to the tissues.
- A high-fibre diet that includes plenty of fruits, vegetables, whole grains, legumes, seeds and nuts is recommended.

Sore throat

This is a symptom indicating that the throat is being invaded by germs.

Spiced mint

> 1 bunch mint
> ½ inch ginger
> 1 orange, peeled
> ½ cup hot water

- Extract the juices, add hot water, and drink immediately.
- Mint eases the soreness in the throat.
- Garlic is a natural antibiotic and ginger is an anti-inflammatory agent.
- Orange has vitamin C, which strengthens the immune system.

- Fresh pineapple juice, a good source of the enzyme bromelain helps in reducing inflammation and is a traditional remedy for sore throat.

Stress

The cause of stress may be emotional, such as worry; biochemical, such as the release of histamine in the tissues in an allergic reaction; or physical, such as illness, injury or over-exertion.

Relaxing drink

  A handful of spinach
  A handful of parsley
  1 clove of garlic
  ¼ inch ginger
  2 carrots
  1 broccoli floweret

- Extract the juices, and mix well.
- Broccoli contains pantothenic acid; ginger, parsley and carrots have zinc; parsley has magnesium; and parsley and spinach have potassium, all of these minerals having to be replenished when they are lost during stress.

- Carrots and parsley are rich in beta-carotene, which is anti-oxidant that helps in protecting the body during stress reactions.
- Garlic and ginger are good sources of blood thinning compounds.
- Cantaloupe is good for the thinning of blood.
- Eat more of fibre-rich foods, as they decrease the cholesterol level that increases during stress.

Thrombosis

It is the blocking of a blood vessel by a blood clot (called a thrombus), which gets formed in the vessel, and if it occurs in an artery leading to an arm or leg, gangrene may set in.

Spicy greens

    A handful of spinach
    1 beet top
    1 green pepper
    1 clove of garlic

- Extract the juices, and mix well.
- Spinach is rich in vitamin B_6, C, E and magnesium, all of which decrease platelet adhesiveness.

- Green pepper is rich in vitamin B_6 and C.
- Beet green is a source of calcium that inhibits platelet adhesiveness.
- Garlic contains selenium that reduces platelet adhesiveness.
- Olive oil, onion, eggplant, melon and pineapple are good anti-coagulants.

Tinnitus

It is a ringing or other noises in the ears, often due only to a build-up of earwax, or may be due to such disorders as Meniere's disease, otitis or other conditions that may lead to deafness.

Cleansing drink

    1 beetroot with leaves

    A handful of parsley

    ½ apple, seeded

    2 carrots

- Extract the juice, and blend well.
- Beetroot and its leaves are potent detoxifiers, and contain manganese.

- Apple is a good source of chromium that helps to correct hypoglycemia by regulating glucose metabolism.
- Carrots have beta-carotene which is a healing nutrient.
- Consume fishes like salmon and mackerel, which are rich in omega-3 fatty acids that improve blood flow in the inner ear.

Ulcers

This is an inflamed, open sore on the skin or on the mucous membrane lining a body cavity.

Cantaloupe shake

    ¼ inch ginger

    ½ cantaloupe

    1 stalk of celery

- Extract the juices, and mix well.
- Cantaloupe is rich in beta-carotene, a healing nutrient.
- Celery helps in healing the ulcer.
- Ginger protects the stomach lining from injury caused by drugs.

- A high-fibre diet consisting of whole grains, fresh fruits and vegetables may help prevent another onset of ulcers.
- Cabbage juice is very soothing, but should not be taken on an empty stomach.

Underweight
This is a condition of being underweight, may be due to genetics, or malnutrition.

Fruity nectar
  ½ papaya

  1 banana

  ½ pineapple

  1 passion fruit, peeled

  ½ cup grapes

  ½ lemon

- Run in a juicer and mix well.
- Papaya is rich in papain, banana in potassium, and pineapple and grapes in bromelain, all of these fruits being natural sources of sugar, boost the calorie levels.
- Lemon is a traditional appetite stimulant.

- Consume complex carbohydrates such as whole grain pasta, potatoes and bananas.

Varicose veins
These are abnormally dilated and knotted blood vessels, fairly close to the surface of the skin, usually in the leg.

Cherry cheer
> 1 cup cherries
> ¼ lime
> 1 bunch green grapes
> 1 slice pineapple

- Extract the juices and mix well.
- Pineapple contains bromelain, which helps in promoting the breakdown of fibroin, and prevents formation of blood clots.
- Cherry is a rich source of anthocyanins as well as proanthocyanins which help to strengthen the venous wall, and also the muscular tone of the vein.
- Eat a high-fibre diet to avoid constipation.
- Increase your intake of ginger, garlic and onion.

Planned Diets

Regular everyday diet
The following diets have be planned for daily use and include the juices mentioned in the previous chapters.

Suggested Menu

Breakfast
> Juice
> Cereal with skim milk
> A piece of fruit
> Wholegrain toast
> Tea

Mid-morning snack
> Juice
> Low cholesterol butter on
> two plain biscuits

Lunch

> Juice
> Vegetable salad
> Bean or pea soup
> 1 sandwich

Evening snack

> Juice
> 1 cup buttermilk

Dinner

> Juice
> Green salad
> Baked potato
> 1 slice brown bread
> ½ serving of seafood

Food groups of the basic diet

- *Cereals, grains, breads, potatoes:* 2-5 servings per meal

  Includes: whole grains such as whole wheat, rye, cornmeal, brown rice; steamed or baked potatoes; low-fat biscuits; whole-wheat pasta and noodles

- *Beans:* 3-5 cups per week for non-vegetarians, and 2-3 cups per day for vegetarians
  Includes: all beans, sprouts, and soya products
- *Nuts and seeds:* 1-2 servings per week
  Includes: all nuts and seeds
- *Vegetables:* 4-8 servings per day
  Includes: all fresh or highly steamed vegetables and fresh vegetables juices
- *Fruits :* 3-5 servings or pieces per day
  Includes: all fresh, raw or cooked fruits, and fruit juices
- *Milk products:* as desired
  Includes: low-fat dairy products, skim milk
- *Meat and poultry:* ½ cup once or twice a week
  Includes: lean meats and white meat
- *Seafood:* 1 cup per day
  Includes: all fish and shellfish
- *Cheese:* not more than 50 gm per day
  Includes: low-fat cheese, low-fat cottage cheese
- *Fats:* 4-7 tbsp per day

Includes: safflower oil, olive oil or flax seed oil

- *Miscellaneous*

  Includes: herbal tea, green or black tea, garlic, ginger, pepper, soya products, low-sugar jams and jellies

Diet for sugar-metabolism disorder – Low-sugar

- The stress here is laid on simple sugars and high in complex carbohydrates.
- This helps in keeping the blood glucose levels balanced and the blood fats low, by slowing down the release of sugar into the bloodstream.
- Always remember to dilute fresh fruit juices and avoid intake of juice on an empty stomach.
- Before embarking on the suggested menus given, consult your doctor.

Suggested Menu

Breakfast
    Juice
    Cereal with skim milk
    Wholegrain toast with ½ tsp butter
    Herbal tea

Mid-morning snack
    Juice
    2 Marie biscuits

Lunch
    Juice
    2 Slices brown bread with non fat butter
        and sprouts
    Green salad with tomatoes

Mid-afternoon snack
    Juice
    Low-fat curd

Evening snack
    Juice
    3 cups popcorn (without butter or oil)

Dinner
>   Juice
>   Pasta or noodles
>   Steamed vegetables
>   1 dry chapatti
>   Green salad

Food groups for inclusion

- *Cereals, grains, breads, potatoes:* 3-6 servings per meal

  Includes: whole grains like brown rice, cornmeal, whole wheat; steamed or baked potatoes; whole wheat pasta and noodles, popcorn

- *Beans:* 5-7 cups per week for non-vegetarians, and 2-3 cups per day for vegetarians

  Includes: all beans, sprouts and soya products

- *Nuts and seeds:* 1-2 servings per week

  Includes: all nuts and seeds

- *Vegetables:* 5-9 servings per day

  Includes: all fresh raw or lightly steamed vegetables, fresh vegetable juices, and carrot juice only with meals

- *Fruit:* 1-3 servings or pieces per week
  Includes: all fresh, raw or cooked fruits eaten whole, all fresh fruit juices diluted with water and drunk with meals
- *Milk products:* as desired
  Includes: low-fat dairy products, skimmed milk, non-fat curd
- *Meat and poultry:* ½ cup once or twice a week
  Includes: lean meats and white meat
- *Seafood :* one cup per day
  Includes: all fish and shellfish
- *Cheese:* 50 gm per day
  Includes: low or non-fat cheese, whole cottage cheese
- *Fats:* 4-7 tsp per day
  Includes: safflower oil, flaxseed oil or olive oil
- *Miscellaneous*
  Includes: herbal tea, black or green tea, garlic, ginger, pepper and soya products

Diet for energising the system immune

- This diet is recommended for those whose immune system is weak.
- During an illness, you may lose vital protein nutrients, and if you are unable to eat solid food, this has to be replenished by high protein juices.
- Eight glasses or more of fluids, in the form of water, juice or soup, should be consumed during the day.
- Since sugar has the tendency to depress the immune system, it is better to avoid sweets.

Suggested Menu

Breakfast
>Juice
>
>½ serving of raw fruit
>
>Wholegrain cereal with non-fat milk
>
>Wholegrain toast
>
>Green or black tea

Mid-morning snack
>Juice
>
>2 Marie biscuits

Lunch
> Juice
> Green salad
> Soup
> Sandwich without butter
> Herbal tea

Mid-afternoon snack
> Juice
> Curd

Evening snack
> Juice

Dinner
> Juice
> Baked cold-water fish
> Steamed vegetables
> Brown rice

Food groups

- *Cereals, grains, breads, potatoes:* 2-5 servings per meal
  Includes: whole grains, wheat germ, bran, steamed or baked potatoes, Marie biscuits,

wheat pasta and noodles, popcorn (oil-less)
- *Beans:* 3-5 cups per week for non-vegetarians, and 2-3 cups per day for vegetarians
  Includes: all beans, sprouts and soya products
- *Nuts and seeds:* 1-2 servings per day
  Includes: all nuts and seeds
- *Vegetables:* 4-8 servings per day
  Includes: all fresh raw or lightly steamed vegetables and juices, especially cabbage, carrot, capsicum and garlic
- *Fruit:* 2-4 servings or pieces per week
  Includes: all fresh fruits or juices, especially apple, pineapple and grapes
- *Milk products:* as desired
  Includes: low-fat dairy products, skimmed milk, non-fat curd
- *Meat and poultry:* No meat, ½ cup poultry product per day
  Includes: white meat
- *Seafood:* 1 cup per day
  Includes: all fish and shellfish, especially cold-water fish such as mackerel and salmon

- *Cheese:* 50 gm per day
  Includes: low or non-fat cheese, low-fat cottage cheese
- *Fats:* 4-7 tsp per day
  Includes: safflower oil, olive oil and flaxseed oil
- *Miscellaneous*
  Includes: herbal tea, water, ginger, garlic, black or green tea (limit to one cup per day)

Find out what you are allergic to

- This diet plan helps you in recognising the foods you are allergic to.
- For a whole week, eat only what has been recommended in the menu – this is the cleansing period.
- Whatever symptoms you may have due to food allergies, should disappear during the cleansing period.
- If symptoms of allergy do not disappear, then you may be allergic to some other factor not related to food.

- The most common foods that one can be allergic to are peach, tea, lamb or sweet potatoes.

- Always seek your doctor's opinion also before you venture out on the recommended diet.

- If you see progress with this diet, you may continue it for another couple of days, but avoid all other foods.

- You may consume the foods in the amount you desire, so that you are not left hungry.

- Once the symptoms disappear, after a week or so, gradually introduce other food items, one at a time.

Suggested Menu

Breakfast

    Apricot or prune juice

    Stewed prunes

    Brown rice cereal with juice (instead of milk

    Brown bread, toasted

    Herbal tea

Lunch

    Baked sweet potato

    Beets or beet greens

    Broiled lamb chop

    Ripe olives

    Peaches

    Herbal tea

Dinner

    Spinach salad with condiments

    Brown rice

    Roast lamb

    Apricots

    Herbal tea

Foods allowed

- *Condiments:* salt and white vinegar
- *Beverages:* herbal tea
- *Cereals and grains:* brown rice, bread made from rice flour
- *Fruits:* apricots, peaches, prunes (cooked), cherries, and ripe olives
- *Fruit juices:* apricot and prune

- *Fats:* cottonseed oil, low-fat margarine, and olive oil
- *Meat:* lamb
- *Vegetables:* sweet potatoes (boiled or baked), beets, beet greens, spinach and lettuce (all thoroughly boiled and seasoned with only allowed condiments and fats)

Diet to detoxify your body
- Children, in their teens, should not follow a strict juice fast.
- Diabetic patients should always consult their doctors before experimenting with their diet.
- Protein powder can be used as a supplement during the fast by those suffering from hypo-glycemia.
- You may fast from one to five days any time of the month.
- Juices of lemon, carrot, cabbage, celery, beets and apple are highly beneficial.
- Include herbal tea, vegetable soups or broth, as well, in your diet.
- You may munch on raw vegetables whenever you feel the need to eat something.

- When you break the fast, ensure that you do not include animal products until the second day after the fast, and then you can include fish and whole grains.

Suggested Menus

Breakfast

You can have any one of the following:
- Juice made from a handful of parsley and 4-6 carrots
- Juice of ¼ inch ginger, 4-5 carrots and ½ apple
- Juice of 1 grapefruit (peeled) and 1 apple
- Juice of 2 peaches, ½ lime, 1 ripe banana and 1 tsp brewer's yeast
- Juice of a handful of parsley, 5 carrots and ½ apple

Mid-morning snack

You can have any one of the following:
- Juice of a handful of spinach, 4 lettuce leaves, 4 sprigs parsley, 6 carrots and ¼ turnip
- Juice of ¼ inch ginger, 1 beet, ½ apple and 4 carrots

- Juice of 1 large cabbage and 2-3 green apples
- Juice of a handful of parsley, ¼ potato, 6 carrots and 1 sprig celery

Lunch

You can have any one of the following:

- Juice of a handful of greens, 3 pineapple slices and 3 radishes
- Juice of 2 parsley sprigs, 4-6 carrots, 2 stalks of celery, 1 apple and ½ beet
- Juice of a handful of parsley and spinach, 4-5 carrots and 2 stalks of celery
- Soup of 2-3 cloves garlic, 1 large tomato, 1 cabbage leaf and 2 stalks of celery

Mid-afternoon snack

You can have any one of the following:

- Juice of ¼ pineapple, ½ apple and ¼ inch ginger
- Juice of a handful of spinach and 4-5 carrots
- juice of a handful of parsley, 5 carrots and ½ apple
- Juice of 1 beet and 2-3 apples

Evening Snack

You can have any one of the following:

- Juice of ½ cantaloupe and 4-5 strawberries
- Juice of 2-inch slice of watermelon and 1 orange segment
- Juice of 1 green apple and 1 stalk of celery
- Juice of 4-6 sprigs of mint leaves, 2 green apples, 1 small wedge of lemon and soda
- Juice of a large bunch of grapes, soda and ½ cup blackberries

Dinner

You can have any one of the following:

- Juice of ½ inch wedge cabbage, 2 green apples and 6 carrots
- Juice of ¼ head cabbage and 3 stalks of celery
- Juice of 3 broccoli flowerets, 1 clove of garlic, 4-5 carrots, 2 stalks of celery and ½ green pepper
- Juice of a handful of parsley, 2-3 cloves of garlic, 3 stalks of celery and 3 carrots
- Juice of 2-3 cloves of garlic, 1 cabbage leaf, 1 large tomato and 2 stalks of celery

Apart from these, you can also have any of the following juices at any time of the day.

Juices of

- ½ cup of blackberries
  1 inch slice of ginger
  1 bunch of green grapes
- 1 large bunch of green grapes
  1 large bunch of red grapes
  1 cup blackberries
- 1 orange, peeled
  1 red apple, seeded
  1 wedge of lime
  1 cup water
- 3 cabbage leaves
  a small handful of parsley
  4-5 carrots
- ¼ inch ginger
  1 apple, seeded
  soda
- 1 small lemon
  soda

When you have completed following the diet to detoxify your body, the following diets, on day one and day two after the fast, may be followed:

Day I

Breakfast
>Juice
>Fruit or vegetable salad with lemon juice dressing
>Herbal tea

Mid-morning snack
>Juice

Lunch
>Juice
>Soup made of garlic, cabbage, tomato and celery
>Vegetable salad with lemon juice dressing

Mid-afternoon snack
>Juice or herbal tea

Dinner
>Juice

Vegetable soup or steamed vegetables

Vegetable salad

Bedtime snack

Juice or herbal tea

Day II

Breakfast

Juice

Fruit or vegetable salad with lemon juice
dressing

Herbal tea

Mid-morning snack

Juice

Lunch

Juice

Vegetable salad

Brown rice

Vegetable soup

Mid-afternoon snack

Juice or herbal tea

Dinner
- Juice
- Vegetable salad, lemon juice and olive oil dressing
- Baked potato
- Baked or broiled fish

Bedtime snack
- Juice or herbal tea

Indian diet for cleansing the system

- This is a diet that is spread over four days.
- The first-day diet is meant to cleanse the colon.
- The second-day diet helps in releasing toxins, excess salts and calcium deposits.
- The third-day diet provides mineral-rich fibre to the digestive tract.
- The final-day diet helps in nourishing the bloodstream, the lymphatic system, and other organs with minerals.

Day I

- Eat only fruits and drink their juice.

- The fruits include apples, pears, berries, melons, peaches and cherries.

Day II
- Drink all the herbal teas that you desire.
- The herbs include peppermint, ginger, chamomile and mint.

Day III
- Eat all the vegetables that you want.
- The vegetables can be raw, steamed or in soup.

Day IV
- Take plenty of vegetable broths.
- The broth may include cauliflower, cabbage, parsley, green pepper, onion, garlic or any other vegetable with salt.

Six-week cleansing diet
- This is designed to help your body in releasing all its toxins gradually, over a period of six weeks.
- During this time, it is recommended that you avoid all animal fats, processed foods and refined products.

- The diet has to be strictly followed for it to be effective.
- You may eat more while you are on this diet because it is low in calories.

Suggested Menu

Breakfast
>   Juice, fresh fruit
>   Cereal with soya milk or juice
>   Wholewheat toast
>   Herbal tea

Mid-morning snack
>   Juice or fresh fruit

Lunch
>   Salad, soup
>   Baked potato
>   Steamed vegetables
>   Herbal tea

Mid-afternoon snack
>   Vegetable juice
>   Carrot slices

Evening snack
    Juice
    Herbal tea
Dinner
    Beans (baked or steamed)
    Salad
    Soup
    Brown rice
    Cooked vegetables
    Fruit
    Herbal tea

Food groups

- *Beverages*: herbal teas
- *Bread and grains*: wholewheat bran, corn, soya, brown rice
- *Cereals*: oats, brown rice, barley, cornmeal
- *Dairy products*: none, except soya milk and soya cheese
- *Fats*: olive oil, safflower oil, sunflower oil, sesame oil, soya oil or corn oil
- *Legumes*: beans, lentils, split peas

- *Vegetables*: all fresh, raw and steamed vegetables, or used in soups, baked or steamed (potatoes in their jackets)
- *Fruit*: fresh fruits, with citrus fruits being used sparingly
- *Juices*: freshly made juices, beet and cabbage especially, 4-6 glasses every day, with more vegetable than fruit juice
- *Nuts*: fresh raw fruits like walnuts and almonds
- *Seeds*: Sesame and pumpkin seeds
- *Sprouts*: all sprouts like lentil, green gram, alfalfa and wheatgrains
- *Desserts*: only fresh fruit or stewed fruit

Diet for reducing weight
- Given below are diet plans for quick weight loss and long-term weight loss.
- The quick weight-loss diet is good for those who need to lose weight only moderately, about 2–13 kg.
- During daytime, drink juice as much as you desire, and have a normal, sensible meal

with your family at night – for quick weight loss.

- These juices are packed with anti-aging nutrients such as vitamin C and beta-carotenes, and hence help you to look younger.
- In case you have symptoms that need a doctor's care, discontinue the diet and seek medical advice.
- If you have any ailments, always consult your doctor before embarking on this diet.

Menu for reducing weight

Breakfast

You can have any one of the following:

- Juice of a handful of parsley and 4-6 carrots
- Juice of 1 grapefruit and 1 apple

Mid-morning snack

You can have any one of the following:

- Juice of ¼ inch of ginger, 4-5 carrots and ½ apple
- Juice of 1 green apple and 1 stalk of celery

Lunch

You can have any one of the following:

- Juice of a handful of parsley and spinach, 4-5 carrots and 2 stalks celery
- Juice of 3 broccoli flowerets, 1 clove of garlic, 4-5 carrots, 2 stalks of celery and ½ green pepper

Mid-afternoon snacks

You can have any one of the following:

- Juice of ¼ inch ginger, 1 beet, ½ apple and 4 carrots
- A handful of greens, 3 pineapple slices and 3 radishes

Evening snack

You can have any one of the following:

- Juice of ½ cantaloupe and 5-6 strawberries
- Juice of 1 green apple and 1 stalk of celery

Dinner

Salad with oil and vinegar dressing, steamed vegetables, brown rice, broiled or baked fish, fruit and herbal tea

Menu for long-term weight reduction

Breakfast

Juice, whole grain bread slice, non-fat curd, green or black tea and an apple

Mid-morning snack

1 apple

Lunch

Juice, vegetable soup, green salad and a slice of wholegrain bread

Evening snack

3 cups popcorn (without fat)

Dinner

Juice, baked skinless chicken, brown rice, yellow vegetables and green vegetables